Paleo Snacks

30+ Paleo Snack Recipes

Table of content

Introduction

I would first like to thank and congratulate you on downloading **"Paleo Snacks: 30+ Paleo Snacks to Satisfy Your Wild Hunger!"** In this book you will find proven steps and strategies on how to make healthy yummy snacks that are considered Paleo. There is a total of 30 delightful Paleo snacks that can be consumed at any time of the day. Just because you are choosing to eat healthier foods does not mean that you have to lose on flavor. These are a collection of healthy Paleo snacks that your loved ones are going to request not because they are healthy, but quite simply because they love how they taste!

Chapter 1- Nutty Paleo Recipes 1-12

1. Mixed Seed Bars

Ingredients:

- one tablespoon of poppy seeds

- five tablespoons of cocoa powder

- twenty fresh dates pitted

- six tablespoons of coconut oil

- one cup of shredded coconut

- five tablespoons of Chia seeds

- half a cup of sunflower seeds

- half a cup of pumpkin seeds

- half a cup of sesame seeds

- two tablespoons of organic honey

Directions:

In a food processor put in Chia seeds, sunflower seeds, shredded coconut, sesame seeds, and pumpkin seeds and process until they are well blended. Set aside. Put the dates, coconut oil, and cocoa powder in the food processor and process until smooth mixture is made. Add a bit of water if necessary. In a bowl mix all ingredients together. Line baking pan with parchment paper and pour the paste on to the baking pan. Spread the paste evenly and smooth out with spatula. Sprinkle top with poppy seeds. Wrap pan with plastic wrap and chill for thirty minutes in fridge. Remove from fridge and cut into desired square sizes. Store in the fridge.

2. *Fruit Quinoa Bars*

Ingredients:

- half a cup of flax seed powder

- half a teaspoon of salt

- half a cup of pomegranate seeds

- half a teaspoon of cinnamon

- half a cup of hemp seeds

- half a cup of sunflower seeds

- half a cup of cooked quinoa

Directions:

Form a paste by putting all the ingredients into a food processor. Line a baking pan with parchment paper. Pour the paste onto it and spread with a spatula. Wrap the baking pan in plastic and place in your freezer overnight. Cut the paste into squares and keep refrigerated.

3. Banana Almond Bars

Ingredients:

- one quarter cup of almonds, chopped

- three eggs

- one cup of almond flour

- three tablespoons of coconut flour

- one quarter cup of coconut oil

- two ripe bananas

- one quarter of a teaspoon of salt

- half a cup of almond butter

Directions:

Mash bananas in a bowl using a fork. Add eggs, salt, coconut flour, coconut oil, almond butter, almond flour and mix well. Lightly grease a baking pan and pour mix into it. Spread evenly with spatula. Top with chopped almonds, press them lightly into mix. Bake in oven at 350° Fahrenheit for 15 minutes. Remove pan from oven and allow to cool. Cut into bars and serve immediately or store in parchment paper in the fridge.

4. *Coco Almond Bars*

Ingredients:

- one tablespoon of organic honey

- half a tablespoon of almond flour

- half a cup of virgin olive oil

- one quarter cup of coconut oil

- one cup of toasted almonds

- half a cup of unsweetened coconut flakes

- one quarter of a teaspoon of sea salt

Directions:

Pulse toasted almonds in food processor until they have a fine texture. Add coconut oil, olive oil, almond flour, honey, salt, coconut flakes and pulse until a paste forms. Line a baking pan with parchment paper and pour paste onto it. Spread evenly with spatula. Put in the fridge for one hour, then remove from fridge and cut into bars, serve immediately or put into plastic container and store in fridge.

5. Roasted Spicy Pecans

Ingredients:

- one tablespoon of water

- one teaspoon of cinnamon

- one egg white

- two cups of pecan halves

- one teaspoon of cayenne pepper

- half a teaspoon of sea salt

- one tablespoon of ground cumin

Directions:

Whisk water and egg white in a bowl until it is foamy. Add cayenne, cumin, cinnamon, salt and pepper and mix well. Add the pecans and fold well to coat them with the egg mixture. Line a baking sheet with parchment paper and grease it with cooking spray. Spread your pecans on baking sheet making sure they are not layered. Put the baking sheet in the oven at 250° Fahrenheit for about 40 minutes. Remove from oven and baking sheet and stir pecans. Return to oven and reduce heat to 200° Fahrenheit for an additional 20 minutes. Remove pecans from baking sheet and allow them to cool. Serve in a bowl or store in an airtight jar.

6. *Sweet Roasted Pecans*

Ingredients:

- one teaspoon of cinnamon

- two cups of pecans

- half a cup of coconut sugar

- one teaspoon of sea salt

- one tablespoon of water

- one egg white

Directions:

Combine in a bowl the salt, cinnamon, and coconut sugar then set aside. In another bowl whisk the egg white and water until they become frothy. Add pecan mix to this and stir making sure to coat pecans well. Add seasoning mixture and combine and coat all the pecans evenly. Line the baking sheet with parchment paper. Place pecans on parchment paper; do not stack them. Put them into oven baking them at 250° Fahrenheit for about one hour. Halfway through the baking process mix pecans around so they will bake evenly. Serve immediately or store in an airtight jar.

7. Roasted Cocoa Almonds

Ingredients:

- two cups of almonds

- two tablespoons of almond flour

- two tablespoons of real maple syrup

- six tablespoons of cocoa powder

Directions:

In a bowl put in almonds and add syrup and mix well to coat the almonds. In another bowl combine cocoa powder and almond flour. Put almonds in cocoa mix and mix well. Line a baking sheet with parchment paper. Grease it lightly with cooking spray. Put almonds on baking sheet to not layer. Bake in oven at 275° Fahrenheit for 20 minutes. Halfway through the baking process stir the almonds so they bake evenly. Allow to cool before serving.

8. *Spicy Roasted Almonds*

Ingredients:

- two cups of almonds

- one tablespoon of organic honey

- three tablespoons of fresh squeezed lime juice

- half a teaspoon of chili powder

- half a teaspoon of cayenne pepper

- one teaspoon of sea salt

Directions:

Whisk the olive oil, lime juice, honey, chili powder, cayenne pepper, and sea salt. Add the almonds and toss to coat. Line a baking sheet with aluminum foil and spray lightly with cooking spray. Lay almonds on baking sheet in one layer. Bake at 350° Fahrenheit for 15 minutes. Remove and mix around almonds then put back into oven for another five minutes. Allow to cool before serving.

9. *Roasted Sweet Cinnamon Walnuts*

Ingredients:

- two cups of walnuts

- half a teaspoon of cinnamon

- one quarter of a cup of coconut sugar

- half a cup of organic honey

- one quarter of a teaspoon of cayenne pepper

- half a teaspoon of sea salt

Directions:

In a saucepan combine cinnamon, coconut sugar, honey, sea salt, and cayenne pepper. Stir well over medium heat until it dissolves, add walnuts and stir well.

Simmer for five minutes until the syrup is browned. Line baking sheet with parchment paper and spray lightly with cooking spray. Spread walnuts on it in one layer. Bake in oven at 180° Fahrenheit for ten minutes. Remove from oven and allow to cool before serving.

10. Herb Roasted Walnuts

Ingredients:

- two cups of walnuts

- one tablespoon of coconut oil

- one quarter teaspoon of salt

- one quarter teaspoon of pepper

- one teaspoon of rosemary, freshly chopped

Directions:

Whisk the rosemary, salt and coconut oil in a bowl. Add the walnuts and toss to coat walnuts. Line a baking sheet with parchment paper. Spread walnuts in one layer on it. Bake in oven 375° Fahrenheit for ten minutes. Stir halfway through and allow to cool before serving.

11. Spicy Sweet Cashews

Ingredients:

- two cups of cashews, halves

- two teaspoons of almond oil

- two tablespoons of coconut sugar

- one quarter teaspoon of paprika

- one quarter teaspoon of sea salt

- one quarter teaspoon of cayenne pepper

Directions:

In a bowl whisk together honey, almond oil, cayenne, paprika and sea salt. Add the cashews and toss to coat them with mixture. Cover a baking sheet with parchment paper and lightly spray with cooking spray. Spread cashews evenly on it in one layer. Sprinkle top of them with coconut sugar. Bake in oven at 350° Fahrenheit for 15 minutes. Remove from oven and stir nuts then put back in oven for another five minutes. Remove from oven and allow to cool before serving or store them in an airtight jar.

12. Roasted Cashews

Ingredients:

- two cups of cashew halves

- one tablespoon of coconut oil

- four tablespoons of organic honey

- one teaspoon of dry mustard

Directions:

Combine in a bowl dry mustard, honey, and coconut oil. Add the cashews and mix to coat them. Put a sheet of aluminum foil on baking sheet and lightly spray with cooking spray. Spread cashews evenly on sheet in one layer. Bake in oven at 350° Fahrenheit for 20 minutes, take out and stir nuts then put back into oven for an additional five minutes. Remove from oven and allow to cool before serving or store in airtight jar.

13. Zucchini Chips

Ingredients:

- one large zucchini

- two eggs, beaten

- half a cup of arrowroot flour

- half a cup of coconut flakes

- one quarter of a teaspoon of pepper

Directions:

Rinse your zucchini and then dry it with a paper towel. Slice it nice and thin. The round slices should be about one quarter of an inch thick or thinner. Dip the zucchini slices first into flour then into eggs with pepper. Dredge slices with coconut flakes. In a pan heat up the oil over medium heat. Fry slices two minutes per side. Fry in batches. Put the cooked zucchini chips in paper towel. Sprinkle with sea salt and serve.

14. Cajun Zucchini Chips

Ingredients:

- one large zucchini

- one cup of fine coconut flakes

- one teaspoon of Cajun seasoning

- six tablespoons of almond milk

- dash of sea salt

Directions:

Rinse zucchini and pat dry with paper towel. Slice into one quarter of an inch rounds set aside. In a bowl combine Cajun seasoning, coconut flakes and dash of salt. Dip zucchini slices in almond milk then into Cajun mix. Press flakes into zucchini so they stick better. Line a baking sheet with aluminum foil and lay zucchini slices in a single layer. Bake in oven at 425° Fahrenheit for 15 minutes. Remove from oven and turn over slices and bake for an additional 15 minutes. Allow the zucchini chips to cool then serve.

15. Coconut Eggplant Fries

Ingredients:

- two eggplants

- half a cup of arrowroot powder

- two cups of fine coconut flakes

- three cups of almond oil

- three eggs, beaten

- salt and pepper one quarter teaspoon of each

Directions:

Rinse your eggplant then dry with a paper towel. Remove the top and bottom parts then cut crosswise into one quarter of an inch circles. Combine arrowroot, eggs, salt and pepper in a bowl. Dip eggplant into mixture and shake off excess. Dredge eggplant in coconut flakes. Heat the almond oil in deep pan over medium heat. Fry eggplant slices two minutes per side in the oil.

16. Eggplant Fries

Ingredients:

- two eggplants

- one cup of pecans, finely chopped

- one tablespoon of parsley, dried

- one quarter of a teaspoon of onion powder

- one quarter of a teaspoon of garlic powder

- one quarter of a teaspoon of cumin

- half a cup of almond milk

- one cup of almond flour

- two tablespoons of apple cider vinegar

- two tablespoons of fresh lemon juice

Directions:

Rinse eggplants and dry with paper towel. Trim off top and bottoms and cut into lengthwise halves. Cut them further into quarters and slice them into half inch thick sticks. In a bowl put almond milk, almond flour, and egg mix well. Add cumin, garlic, paprika, onion, dried parsley, lemon juice, apple cider vinegar. Dip eggplant fries into flour mixture and coat them with chopped pecans. Line a baking sheet with parchment paper and put eggplant fries on it. Bake in oven at 450° Fahrenheit for 10 minutes. Flip eggplant and bake for an additional 10 minutes.

17. Spiced Kale Chips

Ingredients:

- one bunch of kale

- one tablespoon of almond oil

- one quarter of a teaspoon of cayenne pepper

- half a teaspoon of chili powder

- half a teaspoon of onion powder

- half a teaspoon of garlic powder

- one quarter teaspoon of sea salt

Directions:

Remove the stems of the kale leaves and cut them into large pieces. Wash and dry leaves thoroughly. Put kale leaves in a bowl and set aside. In another bowl whisk almond oil, chili powder, paprika, onion powder, salt, and garlic powder. Pour seasoning over the kale leaves. Massage well into the leaves. Line a baking sheet with parchment paper and lay kale leaves on it in a single layer. Bake in oven at 300° Fahrenheit for ten minutes. Flip over kale leaves and bake for an additional ten minutes. Allow to cool before serving.

18. Kale Chips

Ingredients:

- one bunch of kale
- one tablespoon of almond oil
- one quarter teaspoon of pepper
- one quarter teaspoon of sea salt

Directions:

Rinse the kale leaves then dry well. Remove the stems of kale leaves and cut into smaller pieces. Put kale in large bowl and add almond oil, salt and pepper. Lightly massage the kale leaves to coat with seasoning. Line baking sheet with parchment paper and arrange kale leaves on it in single layer. Bake in oven at 300° Fahrenheit for ten minutes, turn kale leaves over and bake for an additional ten minutes. Allow to cool before serving.

19. Cabbage Herb Chips

Ingredients:

- ten green cabbage leaves

- one tablespoon of almond oil

- one tablespoon of rosemary, fresh, chopped

- one quarter teaspoon of salt and pepper each

- two cups of water

- one teaspoon of garlic powder

Directions:

Remove the ribs of the cabbage leaves and cut them into strips about one and a half inches in length. In a pot boil two cups of water and add cabbage. Blanch them until they wilt. Transfer cabbage leaves into a bowl of cold water. Let them stand for five minutes.

Transfer leaves to wire rack so they can dry. In a bowl combine almond oil, garlic powder, sea salt, and pepper. Coat cabbage leaves with oil mixture. Line a baking sheet with parchment paper and place cabbage leaves on it in single layer. Bake in oven at 200° Fahrenheit for about two hours or until the leaves become crispy.

20. *Red Cabbage Chips*

Ingredients:

- 10 red cabbage leaves

- one tablespoon of almond oil

- one quarter teaspoon each of garlic powder, sea salt and pepper

Directions:

Remove the ribs from cabbage leaves and cut them into smaller pieces about two to three inches. Put cabbage in a bowl and set aside. Combine almond oil, garlic powder, sea salt, pepper then pour this over cabbage leaves. Massage lightly into leaves to coat. Line a baking sheet with aluminum foil and arrange leaves on it in a single layer. Bake in oven at 200° Fahrenheit for two hours or until cabbage leaves become crispy. Allow to cool before serving with your favorite dip.

21. Spinach Herb Chips

Ingredients:

- two cups of spinach leaves

- one tablespoon of fresh dill, chopped

- two tablespoons of coconut oil

- one quarter teaspoon of garlic powder

- one quarter teaspoon of salt

- one quarter teaspoon of pepper

Directions:

Combine coconut oil and chopped fresh dill in a bowl. Add spinach and lightly coat with oil mixture. Carefully put spinach leaves on a baking sheet lined with parchment paper. Do not overlap leave put in a single layer. In another bowl combine garlic powder, salt and pepper then sprinkle over top of leaves. Bake in oven at 350° Fahrenheit for ten minutes, flip leaves over and cook for an additional five minutes. Allow to cool before serving.

22. *Spicy Spinach Chips*

Ingredients:

- two cups of spinach leaves

- two tablespoons of olive oil

- one quarter of a teaspoon of sea salt

- one quarter of a teaspoon of cayenne pepper

- one quarter of a teaspoon of paprika

Directions:

Put spinach leaves and olive oil and coat leaves with oil. Take baking sheet and spray it with cooking spray. Arrange leaves in single layer on baking sheet. In a small bowl mix cayenne, paprika, cumin, sea salt, and pepper. Sprinkle this mix on top of leaves. Bake in oven at 350° Fahrenheit for ten minutes. Remove and flip over leaves and bake for an additional ten minutes. Allow to cool before serving.

23. Baked Onion Rings

Ingredients:

- two cups of almond milk
- two large sweet onions
- one cup of almond flour
- one cup of fine coconut flakes
- four egg whites
- half a teaspoon of pepper
- half a teaspoon of sea salt
- half a teaspoon of paprika

Directions:

Peel onions and slice into half inch thick rings. Put them in a bowl and cover with almond milk. Put in fridge for about two hours. Remove onion rings from the fridge and let stand at room temperature for 15 minutes. Beat the egg whites and dip onion rings into it to coat them, dip into coconut flakes. Spray baking sheet with cooking spray, put on onions in single layer. Bake in oven at 425° Fahrenheit for ten minutes, then flip over and bake for an additional ten minutes.

24. Fried Onion Rings

Ingredients:

- two large sweet onions
- one cup of almond milk
- one cup of almond flour
- one egg, beaten
- half a teaspoon of sea salt
- two cups of coconut oil

Directions:

Peel onions and slice into half inch thick rings. Fill a bowl with iced water then submerge onion rings for about one hour. Drain the water and put onion rings in paper towel to absorb excess water. In another bowl whisk together almond milk, sea salt, and beaten egg, slowly add flour and whisk until smooth. Heat oil in deep pan over medium heat. Dip onion rings in the flour mixture than slowly slide them into oil and fry them for five minutes or until golden brown. Put on paper towel to absorb excess oil. Serve on a platter.

25. *Spicy Artichoke Chips*

Ingredients:

- one kilo of artichokes

- one tablespoon of garlic, minced

- one cup of olive oil

- one teaspoon of sea salt

- two tablespoons of thyme, dried

Directions:

Clean your artichokes, remove eyes and rinse well then dry. Slice them into half inch thick slices. In a bowl mix olive oil, thyme, garlic and sea salt. Add the sliced artichoke. Toss around to evenly coat. Line a baking sheet with aluminum foil. Arrange artichokes on baking sheet in single layer. Bake in oven at 175° Fahrenheit for 30 minutes. Remove and flip over and put back in oven for an additional 20 minutes or until tender. Let cool then serve.

26. *Pan Fried Artichoke Chips*

Ingredients:

- one kilo of Jerusalem artichokes

- three tablespoons of fresh parsley, chopped

- six tablespoons of almond oil

- two teaspoons of lemon juice, freshly squeezed

- three tablespoons of sage, fresh, chopped

Directions:

Scrub and rinse artichokes, cut them crosswise to make round chips.   In pan heat two tablespoons of almond oil over medium heat. Put artichokes in pan and fry for five minutes per side. Put fried artichokes on plate and set aside. Add remaining almond oil to pan and add chopped sage. Saute for a minute add lemon juice and stir well. Remove from heat and pour over fried artichokes, toss to coat, top with chopped parsley.

27. Sweet Potato Fries

Ingredients:

- two large sweet potatoes
- two tablespoons of almond oil
- one teaspoon of paprika
- dash of pepper
- dash of sea salt

Directions:

Rinse sweet potatoes and pat dry. Peel skin off potatoes and slice them into half inch strips. Put slices in a bowl of cold water and let stand for ten minutes. Discard the water. Combine the almond oil and paprika, sea salt and pepper then pour over sliced sweet potatoes. Toss to coat. Line baking sheet with aluminum foil add the potatoes in a single layer. Bake in oven at 400° Fahrenheit for 20 minutes. Remove and flip fries over and bake an additional 20 minutes.

28. Steamed Cassava Cake

Ingredients:

- one kilo of cassava

- half a cup of organic honey

- two cups of almond milk

- one quarter of a cup of unsweetened coconut flakes

Directions:

Peel and rinse the cassava well. Use a manual grate to grate the cassava. You can also chop the cassava into chunks then put into the food processor. Process until nice and smooth, set aside. In another bowl, combine almond milk, honey and coconut flakes. Add the cassava to this and stir well. Lightly spray baking pan with cooking spray. Pour the cassava mixture into baking pan and loosely cover with aluminum foil. Put baking pan in a steamer for 20 minutes. Insert a toothpick and if it comes out clean, then the cake is done. Remove the foil and brush some honey on top, sprinkle with coconut flakes. Allow to cool before you serve.

29. Baked Cassava Cake

Ingredients:

- four cups of cassava, grated, drained

- one quarter cup of coconut oil

- half a cup of coconut milk

- one quarter cup of organic honey

- half a teaspoon of sea salt

- three eggs

- one quarter of a cup of fine coconut flakes

Directions:

In a bowl whisk together coconut oil and honey. Add eggs and blend well. Add sea salt and coconut milk and blend well. Fold the coconut flakes into the cassava. Lightly oil baking pan with cooking spray. Pour the cassava mixture into baking pan and bake at 200° Fahrenheit for 40 minutes. You can check to make sure that the cake is done by inserting a toothpick into it. If the toothpick comes out clean your cake is done. Allow the cake to cool before serving.

*30. **Spiced Banana Chips***

Ingredients:

- four unripe bananas

- two tablespoons of almond oil

- one quarter teaspoon of nutmeg

- dash of sea salt

- dash of pepper

Directions:

Peel your bananas and put them in a large pot. Add just enough water to cover the bananas then bring to a boil. Discard the water and allow the bananas to cool. Slice them thinly according to the shape you prefer. In a large bowl combine almond oil, nutmeg, salt, and pepper. Add the bananas and coat them evenly with the mix. Line a baking sheet with parchment paper then spread banana slice in one layer across it. Bake in the oven at 175° Fahrenheit for one hour. Remove from oven and flip over banana slices and cook for an additional hour or until banana slices are crisp. Let them cool before serving.

31. Baked Banana Chips

Ingredients:

- five ripe bananas

- one quarter of a cup of freshly squeezed lemon juice

Directions:

Peel bananas and then cut them crosswise to yield round chips. Use a sharp knife to slice them thin. Put the banana slices in a large bowl and pour the lemon juice over them. Toss them to coat them well. Line baking sheet with parchment paper, put chips on it in single layer. Bake in oven at 200° Fahrenheit for two hours. Remove from oven flip chips over and bake for an additional hour or until they are crisp. Allow to cool before serving.

32. Deep Fried Banana Chips

Ingredients:

- five unripe bananas

- half a cup of cold water

- one cup of almond oil

- one teaspoon of cinnamon

- one cup of pure maple syrup

- one teaspoon of sea salt

Directions:

In a bowl dissolve the sea salt in cold water. Peel bananas and put them in the water for about five minutes. Use a nice sharp knife to slice the bananas lengthwise. Slice them nice and thin. Arrange them on a wire rack and let them dry for 30 minutes. In a deep pan over medium heat add almond oil. Add the banana slices for about two minutes until they are browned. Place cooked banana slices on paper towel to absorb the excess oil. Transfer them to a dish and allow them to cool. In a small pan combine water, maple syrup and cinnamon. Stir until it thickens. Pour syrup over the bananas, toss to coat evenly.

33. Dried Mango Slices

Ingredients:

- two large rip mangoes

Directions:

Rinse mangoes and pat dry. Peel and slice them thinly. Prepare a baking sheet lining it with parchment paper, place mango slices on it in single layer. Bake in oven at 275° Fahrenheit for two hours. Remove and flip over then bake for an additional two hours or until they are dry. Allow the mango slices to cool before serving.

34. Mango Leather

Ingredients:

- three ripe mangoes

Directions:

Rinse mangoes and pat them dry. Slice mango and separate seed and pulp. Put pulp into food processor and puree the mango until smooth. Line a baking sheet with parchment paper, place mango in single layer on it. Spread the puree with spatula and smooth it down. Bake at 200° Fahrenheit for about four hours or until the puree is dry and pliable. Remove from oven and allow to cool. Remove from the parchment paper and cut into strips. Serve or store in airtight jars.

35. Dried Avocado Balls

Ingredients:

- two rip avocados

- two eggs, beaten

- one cup of almond oil

- one small cauliflower head

- one small carrot, chopped finely

- three tablespoons of lemon juice, freshly squeezed

- half a cup of coconut flakes

Directions:

Wash and cut cauliflower into florets. Put them into food processor and process to looks like rice grains. Put into steamer and steam for about five minutes. Process coconut flakes in food processor until they look like crumbs. Cut avocados in half take flesh out and put into bowl. Add lemon juice and carrots mash together until they form a smooth mixture set aside. Spread two tablespoons of cauliflower rice into your palm add one tablespoon of avocado mixture at center. Gently form ball wrapping avocado mixture in rice. Dip balls in egg and roll them in coconut flakes. In a deep pan, heat almond oil and slowly add balls. Fry for two minutes or until the balls turn golden brown. Set cooked balls on paper towel to absorb excess oil and serve warm.

Chapter 4- Paleo Snack Recipes 36-40

36. Fried Avocado

Ingredients:

- two ripe avocados

- two eggs

- one cup of unsweetened coconut flakes

- half a cup of coconut oil

- one quarter of a teaspoon of sea salt

- one quarter cup of coconut flour

Directions:

Put the coconut flakes in food processor and blend until you have fine texture. Combine in a bowl coconut flour with sea salt and set aside. In another bowl beat eggs set aside. Slice avocados into wedges after peeling them. Dip avocado wedges into flour mixture and shake off excess flour. Dip them in the egg and then the coconut flake mix. Heat coconut oil in pan over medium heat and fry until golden brown in color. Put onto paper towel after frying to allow excess oil to be absorbed. Sprinkle avocados with sea salt and serve.

37. ***Grilled Pecans & Peaches***

Ingredients:

- one quarter cup of pecans, chopped

- two tablespoons of almond oil

- one quarter cup of organic honey

- eight fresh peaches

Directions:

Cut peaches into halves and remove the pits. Dip a brush into honey and evenly coat sides of the peaches. Prepare the grill and set it at low-medium heat. Lightly brush grill with almond oil and place peaches on it with the cut side down. Grill them for five minutes and remove from heat and allow to cool. Carefully remove the skin and chop the flesh coarsely and transfer to a plate and drizzle top with honey and top with pecans and serve.

38. Grilled Peaches

Ingredients:

- six fresh peaches

- one quarter of a cup of almond oil

- add cinnamon as garnish

Directions:

Rinse peaches and dry them with paper towel. Cut the peaches into halves and remove the pits. Prepare the grill and set it on medium-low heat. Dip brush in almond oil and carefully brush on peaches. Arrange them on the grill with cut side down. Grill for eight minutes, turn and continue to grill for another five minutes. Brush them throughout about seven times with oil to prevent them from drying out. Let the peaches cool then sprinkle with cinnamon.

39. *Honey Pear Chips*

Ingredients:

- two fresh pairs

- one quarter cup of organic honey

- sprinkle with cocoa powder for garnish

Directions:

Slice your pears very thinly. Line a baking sheet with parchment paper, add pear slices in single layer. Brush top side with honey. Bake in oven at 350° Fahrenheit for about 30 minutes or until the slices are golden brown. Remove from oven and sprinkle with cocoa powder, allow to cool then serve.

40. *Sweet Apple Chips*

Ingredients:

- two green apples

- two cups of water

- one cup of pure maple syrup

- half a cup of lemon juice, freshly squeezed

Directions:

In a small pan combine maple syrup and water mix until it boils. Let simmer for a few minutes then allow to cool. Cut apples crosswise to make round slices. In a bowl drizzle apple slices with lemon. Put apples in syrup and let sit for overnight. Line baking sheet with parchment paper and bake at 200° Fahrenheit for one hour. Flip slices of apple and bake for an additional hour. Serve warm or store in airtight container.

Conclusion

I hope that you and your loved ones will enjoy snacking on this collection of Paleo snacks that are quick and simple to put together. You will feel so much better when you are feeding your family snacks that you know are healthy and offer great flavor at the same time. These are snacks that you can make ahead of time so that they are there throughout the week for your family to easily snack on.

Thanks again for downloading my book I would really appreciate it if you could leave a short review of it at Amazon. It really means a lot to me receiving your positive support of my work—Take Care and Enjoy Your Paleo Snacks!

www.ingramcontent.com/pod-product-compliance
Lightning Source LLC
Chambersburg PA
CBHW050802240726
48654CB00008B/594